Holistic Approach to Male Impotence

Comprehensive Guide for Curing and Reversing Men's Libido Problems with Proven Remedies, Lifestyle Changes, and Natural Strategies to Restore Sexual Performance

Erickson Tom Brown

Copyright

Copyright © 2024 *Erickson Tom Brown.*

Content

Introduction

If you're reading this, it's pretty standard to feel something significant is lacking in your relationship. Even though impotence is common, it can make us feel inadequate because it is characterized by difficulty maintaining a physical connection. The purpose of this book is to let you know that you are not alone and that there is a way to move on, one that can restore your life's strength, connection, and hope. Impotence, commonly referred to as "erectile dysfunction," is the inability to get or keep an erection. It's simply something that can occur for various reasons; it does not indicate weakness or failure. Our physical and emotional energies can be affected by stress, fatigue, health problems, and even everyday routines, which can make intimacy difficult at times. Letting go of the embarrassment or frustration that frequently accompanies this can begin with acknowledging that others also experience it. You can discover new ways to feel powerful and connected; remember, this is a shared experience.

Description

Finding a new path ahead together is the primary goal of this book, which goes beyond simply comprehending impotence. Sometimes, all it takes to recover that delight is a change in perspective. Relationships can be our most significant source of strength and happiness. By concentrating on the whole person—body, mind, and emotions—we will examine how to overcome these obstacles. By reviewing all the aspects of ourselves and our relationship that contribute to genuine connection, this "holistic" approach will help us realize that a healthier relationship is not the result of a single quick fix. This book will lead you to a place of healing, understanding, and rekindled intimacy through easy, practical methods. You and your spouse can discover new ways to support one another and embrace this journey by reading, thinking about, and putting the ideas here into practice. This is a start—an opportunity to feel empowered and hopeful as you go together from adversity to strength.

CHAPTER 1

Everyone wants to feel intimate and connected in a relationship. However, impotence, commonly known as erectile dysfunction (ED), is one of the difficulties that occasionally arise that we do not anticipate. This chapter will clarify some common misconceptions and examine the definition and causes of impotence. The intention is to assist you in realizing that impotence is a familiar feeling that can be addressed with compassion, empathy, and support rather than defining you or your relationship.

What is Impotence?

A person who struggles to get or maintain an erection that is hard enough for sexual activity is said to have impotence. It is merely a physical difficulty that many encounter at some point; it does not imply anything "wrong" with them. Some people may experience it sporadically, sometimes during times of stress, exhaustion, or even anxiety.

For others, it might be a more frequent sensation. It might cause feelings of disappointment, annoyance, or even embarrassment when it occurs repeatedly. However, it's crucial to keep in mind that impotence is widespread. Millions of men worldwide are said to suffer from erectile dysfunction in some capacity. Therefore, you are certainly not alone if you or your partner are experiencing this. A person's feelings about themselves and their relationship can be impacted by impotence, which is frequently more than just a physical condition. Finding answers and advancing together, however, can be significantly aided by acknowledging it for what it is: a condition that can be controlled.

Why Men Experience Impotence

Knowing the many causes of impotence can help relieve some of the stress you may be experiencing. Physical causes and mental or emotional causes are the two primary causes. Erection problems are frequently caused by multiple factors rather than a single cause.

1. **Physical Factors**:
The body greatly influences sexual health, and erections can be affected by several physical variables. Blood flow and circulation: When blood enters the penis, it fills it and gives it rigidity, resulting in erections. Therefore, any medical condition that impacts blood flow, such as diabetes, high blood pressure, or heart disease, might make erections more difficult. It might be challenging to achieve or maintain an erection when blood flow is poor.

- **Hormones**

Hormones, particularly testosterone, are essential for sexual desire and health. Low hormone levels can impact a person's energy, mood, and longing for closeness. Age-related hormonal changes are regular, but they can also occasionally impact erections.

- **Drugs**

Some drugs, particularly those for anxiety, depression, or high blood pressure, might have adverse consequences that affect a person's sexual health. It's wise to consult a doctor if you're taking medicine and observe changes in your erections. They might modify your treatment or suggest alternative options. Erections can also be impacted by lifestyle factors, such as smoking, binge drinking, or eating a diet heavy in sweets and harmful fats. Erections may become more challenging due to these behaviors that disrupt blood flow and general wellness.

- **Rest and Sleep**

Sleep is essential for energy and general well-being. Poor sleep or illnesses like sleep apnea, a disease in which breathing stops and begins while one sleeps, can cause fatigue and a lack of interest in or energy for intimacy.

2. Emotional and Mental Factors:

The leading cause of impotence can occasionally be found in the mind. Because sexual health and mental and emotional well-being are firmly related, our bodies may not react as well if we are experiencing anxiety, stress, or depression.

- **Stress**

Our bodies release cortisol and other hormones when we are under stress, which can interfere with other hormones and make it difficult to feel at ease or interested in intimacy. Stress also has an impact on our eating habits, sleep patterns, and even interpersonal communication, all of which can affect our sexual health.

- **Anxiety**

Anxiety is a state of concern or uneasiness that can consume a significant amount of mental energy. Some people experience a cycle of impotence that increases the likelihood that they will experience it again due to anxiety about sexual performance or concerns about whether they can satisfy their spouse. This is frequently referred to as "performance anxiety."

- **Depression**

Depression is more than just sadness; it can also result in poor energy, a loss of interest in activities we formerly enjoyed, and a loss of interpersonal relationships. Erectile dysfunction may result from depression's effects on the brain chemicals that give us pleasure.

Relationship Concerns

Unresolved disputes or problems in a partnership may impact intimacy. Perhaps the partnership has gone through a difficult period, or there is a sense of separation or unresolved dispute.

Impotence risk can be decreased, and closeness can be significantly enhanced by addressing these issues.

Dispelling Myths Regarding Impotence

Impotence is the subject of numerous myths, which can occasionally cause embarrassment or anxiety. We can lessen the emotional burden that impotence can cause by being aware of what it is and is not. Let's examine some prevalent myths:

Myth 1

Impotence is a Sign of Inadequate Masculinity. This is not accurate at all. Self-worth and masculinity are unrelated to impotence. Many guys suffer from this medical ailment. It doesn't define you, just as other health issues do. Keep in mind that it's a familiar sensation that occurs for a variety of causes.

Myth 2

Impotence Is Not Exclusive to the Elderly Although age can be a factor, impotence can also affect younger people. Lifestyle choices, stress, or medical issues can impact anyone, regardless of age. Impotence is common for younger men, particularly at stressful moments in their lives.

Myth 3

You Are the Only One with Impotence is not "in your head," even though mental and emotional well-being may be a factor. A combination of cognitive, emotional, and physical components are frequently involved. People may believe that it's their responsibility if it's dismissed as solely mental, even though there are generally other contributing factors.

Myth 4

If something occurs once, it will always happen, but impotence doesn't need to last forever. Some people may only experience it occasionally, perhaps due to stress, exhaustion, or other circumstances. Others may have it more frequently, but it's still tolerable. Numerous methods and therapies can be beneficial.

Myth 5

Discussing It Will Make It Worse In actuality, having an honest and open conversation with a spouse can reduce stress and strengthen the bond between the two of you. It fosters understanding and might lessen tension or concerns about criticism. Moving forward as a team frequently requires effective communication. The first step in overcoming impotence is comprehending it and its causes. The goal of this trip is to strengthen your relationship with your partner and yourself, not to be flawless.

Chapter 2

How Impotence Affects Our Relationships

The basis of relationships is intimacy, trust, and connection; however, impotence can upend these fundamental tenets. Impotence is more than just a medical problem for many couples; it's an emotional one that can cause discontent, anger, and even miscommunication. In this chapter, we'll examine how impotence can impact a couple and their relationship. We'll also explore the benefits of communication, including how it can foster empathy, understanding, and the opportunity to develop a closer bond through open dialogue.

Emotions and Dissatisfactions

When impotence strikes, a variety of feelings are frequently present. Although the feelings of each individual in the relationship may differ, they are genuine and legitimate for all parties. Let's examine some of the most typical human emotions and their causes.

1. **Anger and Disillusionment**:
The impotent person may feel an intense sense of frustration. They may be disappointed that they can't communicate intimacy the way they'd like to or feel as though their body isn't cooperating. This annoyance may also affect their self-perception; even though impotence is merely a condition and not a reflection of their value, they may feel they are not performing their function as a partner.

Although it could manifest differently, the partner may also experience frustration. They may be perplexed as to why the connection has changed or uncertain what is happening. Even when it's not the case, they can question whether they're to blame or whether their partner is losing interest. These ideas can easily be left unsaid, which leads to tension and further annoyance.

2. **Sadness and Loss:**
It's normal to feel depressed when something as intimate is disturbed. This melancholy may result from a sense of

loss—a loss of intimacy, confidence, or even the way things used to be. Some people who experience impotence may feel less attractive or fear that their spouse may have a different opinion of them.

It's acceptable and reasonable to experience sadness, but it's also critical to realize that it need not last forever. With the correct understanding and support, it is possible to transform this melancholy into a chance to re-establish intimacy in novel ways.

3. **Fear and Concern:**

The fear that things will never get better or that the relationship will be permanently altered might result from impotence. Both couples can be concerned that their intimacy will never recover or that it will impact their feelings for one another down the road. If this concern is not addressed, it can occasionally cause distance since the two parties may begin to remove themselves rather than confront the problem jointly.

4. **Guilt and Shame**:

Many people feel shame when impotent as if they are somehow to blame for something out of their control. Because they may feel judged or afraid of disappointing their spouse, this shame can make it hard for them to be honest and open.

Another factor may be guilt; the impotent person may feel they are failing their spouse, and the partner may feel bad for being angry or let down. Although these feelings—sadness, anxiety, humiliation, and frustration—are normal, they don't have to rule the relationship.

Couples can experience these emotions together and find strength in one another's support if they communicate, are compassionate, and understand.

Importance of Communication

One of the most effective ways to mend during irritation or despair is to have an honest conversation with one another. Communication fosters a secure environment where both partners may express their emotions, concerns, and aspirations despite the initial discomfort. Understanding one another's wants, needs, and anxieties through open communication is crucial for establishing a foundation of empathy and trust.

1. **Starting the Discussion**: Starting a talk regarding impotence can be challenging, but remember that being open is a sign of love

and bravery. Expressing your feelings gently and blame-freely is one approach to start.

For instance, saying something like, "I wanted to share what's on my mind because I've been feeling a little down about our intimacy lately," allows for a calm and honest talk. It's also crucial for the spouse to address the subject with empathy. "I understand that things have been difficult lately, and I'm here to support you," you might add. How can we resolve this as a team?

This communicates to your partner that you support them and are on the same page.

2. **Empathy and Active Listening:** An essential component of communication is listening. Listening to one partner's feelings is critical without interjecting or drawing conclusions too quickly. Give each other room to discuss your mind and try to comprehend their perspectives. You can feel appreciated and understood by demonstrating empathy or putting yourself in the other person's shoes. For example, when one partner expresses shame, the other can reassure them by saying, "I don't see you any differently because of this." Sayings like "We're in this together"

might help dispel guilt by demonstrating that love and acceptance are still present in the partnership.

3. **Resolving Misconceptions and Fears**
Impotence might occasionally raise misconceptions or anxieties, but discussing these issues honestly can help keep them from becoming obstacles. Both partners can resolve any misconceptions if one partner expresses concern that the other may be losing interest. Hearing statements such as "My feelings for you haven't changed at all" might be comforting. Our relationship is really important to me, so I want to work through this. By addressing fears together, a couple can feel more secure and enhance their relationship.

4. **Emphasizing Emotional Closeness**: Emotional closeness can grow stronger during this period, even though physical intimacy may be impacted. Spending quality time together, sharing everyday experiences, and expressing affection can all make both couples feel important and connected. Feeling more connected on a deeper level is the goal of emotional intimacy, which can improve a relationship's warmth, trust, and happiness.

Both partners can be reminded of their proximity by concentrating on tiny gestures of affection, such as holding hands, giving hugs, or just spending time discussing topics you both enjoy. This emotional connection frequently serves as the cornerstone that enables couples to advance and forge an even closer bond.

4. **Together, we are able to find solutions**

It's simpler to talk about possible solutions if you've established open communication. You might want to try some lifestyle modifications collectively, such as taking walks, learning relaxation techniques, or getting medical advice as a group. Finding answers jointly gives both parties the impression that they are actively trying to get well, which fosters a sense of hope and partnership. Relationship distance doesn't have to result from impotence. Rather, it can be a chance to get to know one another better, to be honest and vulnerable, and to develop a closer, more sympathetic bond. Honest emotional expression between partners is made possible by communication, which makes both parties feel heard, appreciated, and respected. Recall that the goal of this journey is to grow together and encourage one another through the difficulties, not to achieve perfection. One step at a time, couples can transition from frustration to understanding and from difficulty to strength by maintaining open lines of communication.

CHAPTER 3

The Power of a Holistic Approach to Impotence

It's simple to concentrate on a single remedy, like exercise or medical intervention, when considering how to overcome obstacles like impotence. But occasionally, one strategy is insufficient to address all of the causes of the conflict. A holistic approach a method of caring for the full person rather than just one aspect comes into play here. Because the body, mind, and emotions are interconnected and function as a single unit, holistic health refers to treating them all at once. We'll examine what "holistic" actually means in this chapter and why it can have an impact. We'll explore how our mental, emotional, and physical well-being are interconnected and how making minor adjustments in each can eventually result in significant changes.

What Is Holistic?

The concept of "whole" considering all the components that comprise an individual is where the word "holistic" originates. Focussing on a person's physical, mental, and emotional well-being is known as holistic health. A holistic approach to issues like impotence considers mental and emotional well-being in addition to physical health (such as blood flow or hormones) and physical health (such as stress or worry) (such as feelings of connection and intimacy with a partner). A holistic approach seeks to promote balance and well-being by attending to each of these areas, which will enable one to confront obstacles like impotence with a refreshed sense of vigour.

Three Importance of Holistic Health

1. Body
The state of our heart, blood vessels, muscles, and hormones is referred to as our body. Exercise, nutrition, rest, and medical assistance are all ways to enhance physical health. More vitality, improved circulation, and increased stress tolerance are all characteristics of a healthy body that can support intimacy and connection.

2. **Mind**

This refers to our mental well-being, encompassing our concentration, thinking, and stress management techniques. Our thoughts have an impact on how we perceive and respond to difficulties. For instance, a person's body may also be impacted by a mental block brought on by anxiety or worry. We can feel more relaxed and manage stress by engaging in techniques like deep breathing, mindfulness, and meditation.

3. **Heart**

In this context, "heart" refers to our feelings and connections. How we feel about ourselves and our spouse is greatly influenced by how we feel connected, loved, and respected. We feel closer and find it simpler to deal with challenges as a team when we feel comfortable being open and vulnerable. Positive communication, empathy, and expressing gratitude enhance our hearts, or emotional wellness.

How the Mind, Heart and Body Interact with Each Other

Understanding that the body, mind, and heart are interconnected and have an impact on one another is essential to adopting a holistic approach.

Let's examine how they cooperate and how taking care of each component can help people overcome obstacles like impotence.

1. **How the Body Function**:

The basis of our general health is our body. We feel stronger, more capable, and have more energy when we take care of our physical health. Numerous aspects of physical health, such as muscle strength, hormone balance, and blood circulation, can enhance intimacy. Here are some benefits of taking care of the body:

- **Exercise**

One of the most effective ways to enhance physical health is through exercise. Regular exercise improves the heart's ability to pump blood, which is crucial for sustaining powerful erections. Endorphins, sometimes referred to as "feel-good" hormones, are released during exercise and have the ability to improve mood and reduce stress.

- **Healthy Eating**

Our bodies are powered by the food we eat. Maintaining energy, supporting hormones, and enhancing blood flow can all be achieved by eating balanced meals full of fruits, vegetables, lean meats, and healthy fats. A balanced diet also promotes emotional stability and mental clarity.

- **Sleep**

The body needs quality sleep in order to recover and heal. We are more alert, more focused, and better able to manage stress when we get enough sleep. Hormone balance, which affects both physical and mental health, is another benefit of sleep. By putting our physical health first, we build a strong foundation for our mental and emotional well-being.

2. How the Mind Function:

How we handle difficulties is greatly influenced by our mental state, or mental health. Our physical and emotional well-being is influenced by our beliefs, stress, and thoughts. The body's capacity to relax can be hampered by stress or anxiety, which can have an impact on hormone levels, blood flow, and sleep.

- **Handling Stress**

Prolonged stress can strain the body and the mind. In addition to raising emotions of annoyance or despair, it can result in health problems like elevated blood pressure. These effects can be lessened by using stress management techniques including deep breathing, meditation, or simply taking some time to unwind.

- **Positive Thinking**

Our perceptions of ourselves and our circumstances can significantly influence our actions. A cheerful attitude lessens fear and fosters hope when we face obstacles. This does not include acting as though everything is flawless, but rather concentrating on areas for improvement and acknowledging minor victories.

- **Relaxation and mindfulness**

Being completely present in the moment without passing judgement is known as mindfulness, and it can help the mind feel more at ease. Being aware makes it simpler to feel at ease and receptive to good experiences since we are less preoccupied with fears about the future or previous mistakes. Taking care of our mental health entails allowing ourselves the time and space to think and cope with stress, which improves the body-emotional connection.

3. **The Heart's Function:**

Heart health, often known as emotional health, is about our relationships with others and ourselves. Feeling emotionally connected and supported in relationships can have a significant impact on our physical and mental well-being.

A safe environment is created where both partners can confront difficulties jointly when they feel appreciated, accepted, and understood. Bonding and Connection: Being emotionally and physically there for one another is a key component of emotional connection. Being so close fosters trust, which makes it simpler to discuss challenging subjects like impotence without fear of condemnation or embarrassment.

- **Expressing Gratitude**

Even in tiny ways, expressing gratitude strengthens the relationship's favourable emotions. Reminding both partners that they are loved and appreciated can be accomplished by saying "thank you," sharing words of support, or spending quality time together.

- **Patience and Empathy**

Empathy entails understanding your partner's emotions and placing yourself in their position. Being patient is giving one another the space and time to resolve conflicts without feeling rushed. As you both collaborate to find answers, these traits can allay fears and foster a sense of solidarity.

Relationships are strengthened when we take care of our emotional well-being because it creates room for understanding, support, and the sense that we are "in this together."

Bringing Everything Together

Taking a comprehensive approach to impotence means considering the big picture. In addition to treating the illness directly, taking care of our bodies, minds, and emotions lays the groundwork for a happy and healthy relationship. Each component mental tranquilly, emotional intimacy, and physical health supports the others, generating a cycle of well-being that might facilitate overcoming obstacles and fostering a closer bond with our spouse.

Building habits and making decisions that support the full person are the goals of holistic health, not finding fast fixes. Couples can go from difficulty to strength by taking care of their bodies, calming their minds, and nourishing their hearts. They will realise that they are stronger and more resilient together. The goal of this journey is to embrace every aspect of who we are and our relationship while forging a future based on love, care, and balance.

Chapter 4

How Regain Your Physical Health

One of the most important steps in conquering impotence and fortifying the body is restoring physical health. Our confidence is increased and the groundwork for our mental and emotional health is laid when we feel physically strong and invigorated. This chapter will discuss some easy ways to enhance physical health by emphasizing three key areas: rest, exercise, and a good diet. These procedures don't need to be laborious or difficult. A stronger, healthier, and more resilient body can be achieved by making little, regular changes over time.

Eat Healthy

Providing Your Body with Fuel Our energy, concentration, and general health are all directly impacted by the foods we eat. A healthy diet is about selecting foods that boost your energy levels, enhance blood circulation, and support your body's natural functions—it's not about eliminating everything you enjoy. Here are some easy steps to start eating in a way that supports intimacy and fuels your body.

1. **Eat Lots of Vegetables and Fruits**

Vitamins, minerals, and antioxidants found in abundance in fruits and vegetables support the body's defences against stress, increase immunity, and preserve normal blood flow. Berries are high in antioxidants that shield the body's cells, while other fruits, such as avocados and bananas, include potassium, which aids in blood circulation. Aim to have half of your plate full of vibrant fruits and veggies. You may be sure you're getting a diverse assortment of nutrients by eating foods of different colours.

2. **Go for Lean Proteins**

Energy and muscle strength depend on protein. Fish, poultry, beans, and nuts are examples of lean proteins that give the body the building blocks it needs for development and repair. Omega-3 fatty acids, which promote circulation and heart health, are also abundant in fish, particularly fatty fish like salmon and mackerel.

To maintain consistent energy levels, include a source of lean protein with every meal. Try plant-based proteins like tofu, lentils, and beans if you don't consume meat.

3. **Add Whole Grains to your Diet**

Whole grains that are high in fibre and give you sustained energy include quinoa, brown rice, and oats. Whole grains, as opposed to refined grains, lessen energy dips by assisting in maintaining stable blood sugar levels. Additionally, they promote heart health, which is essential for sustaining blood flow and endurance. Advice: Consider using whole-grain pasta or bread instead of white ones. They will provide you additional nutrients and prolong the sense of fullness.

4. **Good Fats are your Best Friends**

Not every fat is harmful. Hormone production and brain health depend on healthy fats, such as those in avocados, nuts, seeds, and olive oil. These fats sustain the body's natural functions by giving it a consistent supply of energy and assisting in the maintenance of hormone balance. Include a little portion of healthy fat in meals, such as an avocado slice or a handful of almonds. Additionally, healthy fats can increase satisfaction by giving meals a sense of completion.

5. **Take Lots of water**

Water is necessary for nearly all body processes. Maintaining hydration aids digestion, boosts energy levels, and enhances attention. Fatigue brought on by dehydration might make it more difficult to feel alert and active. Try to consume six to eight glasses of water each day. If you don't like the taste of plain water, try adding a slice of cucumber or lemon. You can significantly enhance your mood by making tiny, incremental dietary modifications.

Recall that balance, not perfection, is the key to healthy eating. Eat nutrient-dense foods to nourish your body and indulge in your favourite sweets in moderation.

The Importance of Exercise:

In addition to enhancing physical health, regular exercise can raise energy levels, mood, and confidence. Simple, regular workouts can have an impact; a complex regimen is not necessary to begin seeing results. Now let's examine some simple fitness routines that can help boost confidence and strength.

- **Strolling**

Walking is a fantastic low-impact workout that increases heart strength, circulation, and vitality. It's also an easy method of stress relief and mental clarity. Even 20 to

30 minutes a day can have a significant impact on your health.

Advice:
To start your day with vigour, try taking a little stroll in the morning or after meals. Consider utilising a treadmill or simply walking in place indoors if you are unable to stroll outside.

- **Exercises**

Using Your Bodyweight Without the use of any equipment, bodyweight workouts such as push-ups, lunges, and squats can assist increase strength. Major muscular groups are worked by these workouts, which can improve general fitness and endurance. As your strength increases, progressively increase the number of repetitions you begin with.

Advice:
Start with easy sets, such as ten lunges or ten squats, then increase as you get more powerful. To prevent injury, concentrate on form.

- **Flexibility and Stretching:**

Stretching encourages relaxation, eases tense muscles, and increases flexibility. Additionally, stretching gently can increase blood flow and lower stress levels, which makes it simpler to maintain an active lifestyle. A few minutes of stretching in the morning or after working out is a good idea. Pay attention to your back, arms, and legs, which are your main muscle groups.

- **Breathing Deeply and Moving Mindfully**

Breathing-based exercises, such as yoga and tai chi, are beneficial for mental and physical strength. These activities promote awareness, which lowers stress and promotes relaxation.

Advice:
Begin with a quick stretching exercise or a few deep breaths. Energy levels can be raised and the mind calmed in as little as five minutes. Exercise doesn't have to be time-consuming or strenuous. A well-rounded regimen that promotes physical health and increases confidence can be created by combining stretching, weight training, and mild aerobics. Consistency is essential; little daily efforts build up over time.

- **Rest and Recuperation**:

The Influence of Sound Sleep Despite being frequently disregarded, sleep is essential for both mental and physical well-being. A restful night's sleep boosts energy, enhances concentration, and aids in the body's healing process. It's simpler to manage stress, maintain an active lifestyle, and take pleasure in our everyday activities when we get enough sleep.

How to Improve your sex Life by 65% Through Sleep

1. Sleep 7-9 Hours Dialy

The body repairs cells, balances hormones, and calms the mind while we sleep. The body cannot function at its peak when sleep is insufficient, which results in exhaustion, depression, and decreased motivation. Sleep is crucial for immune system performance, muscle repair, and general vitality. Try to get between 7 and 9 hours of sleep per night. Sleeping regularly facilitates the regulation of the body's natural rhythm, which makes it simpler to awaken feeling rejuvenated.

2. Establishing a Calm Nighttime

Routine The body can be told its time to wind down with a soothing sleep routine. Deep breathing exercises, relaxing music, and reading can all help the mind unwind and be ready for sleep. Steer clear of bright lights and screens as they can disrupt the body's normal sleep signals.

Advice:
Try establishing a consistent bedtime and winding down half an hour before bed. It may be simpler to fall asleep and remain asleep through the night if you are consistent.

3. **Reducing Heavy Meals and Caffeine:**

Heavy meals right before bed and caffeine can interfere with sleep. It can be challenging to settle in after a large lunch because caffeine remains in the bloodstream for hours. If you're hungry, go for a light snack instead, such as a small piece of fruit.

Advice:
Aim to eat your final meal two to three hours before bed, and steer clear of caffeine after noon. This aids the body in getting ready for a good night's sleep.

4. **Creating a Sleep Environment That Is Comfortable**:

The quality of your sleep is greatly influenced by your sleeping environment. A quiet, dark, and chilly environment promotes relaxation and deep sleep. If necessary, think about utilising earphones, a fan, or blackout curtains.

Advice:
Make your bedroom a sleep-friendly place by clearing all distractions and designating it as such. This makes it easier for your mind to connect the space with rest and sleep. Regular exercise, a healthy diet, and adequate sleep all contribute to physical well-being. We go closer to feeling invigorated, self-assured, and prepared to savour life's moments with every step we take to improve our bodies.

Chapter 5

Emotional control among partners can foster intimacy and understanding that fortifies the connection in any relationship. Emotions can run high while facing difficulties like impotence, and tension, anxiety, and even annoyance can make things seem more difficult. However, by working together to learn how to control our emotions, we can transform these trying times into chances for development and bonding. Three crucial facets of managing emotions as a pair will be covered in this chapter: managing stress, encouraging one another's emotions, and keeping an optimistic outlook. Together, you can build a solid emotional support system that will enable you to overcome any obstacle as a team.

Together We all encounter stress, which can make even minor difficulties seem insurmountable. Stress can have an impact on our relationships with one another as well as our emotional states. A peaceful and encouraging atmosphere can be created for both parties by learning stress management techniques.

1. **Deep Breathing and Relaxation**:
One of the easiest strategies to deal with stress is to practise deep breathing. Breathing deeply and slowly tells the body that it's time to relax, which can drop heart rate, ease tension, and promote mental calmness. Even a brief period of time spent practicing deep breathing together can foster a sense of relaxation and tranquilly. Do a quick breathing technique with each other. Close your eyes, find a quiet place to sit, and inhale deeply and slowly through your nose. Hold the breath for a few seconds, then let it slowly through your mouth. Continue until both of you feel more at ease, or for five breaths.

2. **Having Fun with Hobbies:**
One of the best ways to reduce stress and create happy memories is to have fun together. Taking part in a pastime, such as

cooking, gardening, or sports, provides a respite from everyday concerns and enables you to have fun together. Anything that you both enjoy can make you happy and reduce stress, so hobbies don't have to be difficult or time-consuming. Pick a pastime that you both can like, such as going on a nature walk or preparing a new dish. Reconnecting and relieving stress can be achieved by sharing these little moments.

3. **Taking pauses and engaging in self-care**:

It's acceptable to take a break when tension begins to rise. Whether it's sipping tea, reading a favourite book, or just spending some quiet time, self-care entails making time to rejuvenate. You might come back to the connection feeling rejuvenated and prepared to listen or share after taking a few minutes to yourself. Remind one another to take pauses as necessary. Self-care is not selfish; rather, it's a means of ensuring that you both have the stamina and composure to tackle obstacles together. You may create a space where both partners feel supported and prepared to face each day with ease and serenity by figuring out how to deal with stress as a pair.

How to Encourage One Another's Emotions

Being there to listen, comprehend, and provide consolation is just as important as fixing each other's difficulties. Trust is increased and a secure environment for open communication is created when both sides feel heard and appreciated. Supporting one another's emotions fosters togetherness and makes overcoming obstacles as a team easier.

1. Listening Without Making Any Judgements:

One of the easiest yet most effective ways to offer help is to listen. It can be tempting to provide counsel when one spouse is expressing their emotions, but most of the time, listening is all that is required. It makes your spouse feel valued and comfortable to give them the freedom to express themselves without fear of criticism. Show that you are paying attention by nodding or gently acknowledging what they are saying. This is known as "active listening." Use expressions like "Thank you for sharing this with me" or "I understand how that must feel" to demonstrate empathy.

2. Demonstrating Empathy:

Putting oneself in your partner's position is a sign of empathy. You acknowledge their emotions and validate their experience when you can empathise with one another. This just demonstrates that you're attempting to comprehend their viewpoint; it doesn't imply that you have to agree with anything they have to say. Make an effort to react empathetically to your partner's emotions. Give them a helpful response, such as "I'm here for you" or "Let's get through this together," and acknowledge that it's acceptable for them to feel stressed.

3. Providing Comfort

Difficulties might lead to periods of uncertainty or anxiety. In order to remind each other that you are in this together and that better times are coming, it can be very helpful to offer reassurance. Simple acts of kindness, such as holding hands, giving a reassuring embrace, or saying a few encouraging words, can improve the relationship and offer emotional stability. A few easy sentences that can help you reaffirm your commitment to supporting each other are "I believe in us," "We'll find a way through this," and "You're not alone."

It is not necessary to "fix" everything in order to support one another's sentiments; rather, it is about establishing a secure and reassuring environment where both partners feel appreciated, acknowledged, and seen.

The Function of a Positive Attitude

Concentrating on Better Times to Come A positive outlook might assist in reorienting attention from concerns and difficulties to opportunities and hope. When both partners make an effort to maintain a positive attitude, it fosters a resilient and hopeful environment that can significantly impact difficult times.

1. **Always Show an Act of Gratitude**:
Being grateful entails valuing all of life's blessings, no matter how minor. Couples can cultivate a sense of joy and appreciation by practicing thankfulness, which can help them change their focus from what is lacking to what is functioning well. You might thank each other for your shared moments, strengths, and support. Try sharing one thing for which you are thankful at the beginning or conclusion of each day. Both spouses can benefit from maintaining a positive mentality by adopting this modest habit.

2. **Put Progress Above Perfection:**
Sometimes difficulties can make it simple to concentrate on what is "wrong" or not functioning flawlessly. However, you can foster a sense of advancement and success by concentrating on little victories rather than perfection. Acknowledging even small progress can enhance spirits and give both parties optimism. Advice: Whether it's a brief moment of laughing, a constructive discussion, or a minor advancement in connection or health, celebrate little victories with each other. Every advancement, no matter how tiny, is an indication of development.

3. **Together, we set constructive goals:**
Establishing objectives provides both parties with something to strive for and anticipate. These objectives don't have to be lofty; they can be as straightforward as organizing a night out, scheduling time for a common pastime, or developing a self-care regimen. Positivity fosters a feeling of purpose and provides motivation for both partners to continue their journey together. Pick a goal that has personal significance for you both, such as exploring a new activity together or engaging in a daily routine like a relaxation technique or a moment of thankfulness.

As a team, setting and accomplishing goals generates great momentum and memories.

4. **Imagining Better Times to Come:**
A useful technique that can keep both parties inspired and upbeat is visualisation. By imagining a happy, intimate, and healthy future, you both produce a positive image that serves as a reminder of your goals. This optimistic outlook can improve the quality of each day and promote perseverance in the face of adversity. Spend some time together envisioning a happy future, including how you will feel, what you will do, and how you will continue to help one another. You may foster a sense of hope among people by imagining better times ahead, which helps make difficulties seem transient and doable.

Accepting the Path Together

A key component of overcoming obstacles in life as a team is managing emotions collectively. You build a solid emotional foundation that keeps you resilient and linked by dealing with stress, encouraging one another's emotions, and maintaining an optimistic mindset. Together, these little actions build a partnership based on mutual respect, trust, and hope. Remember that it's acceptable to experience ups and downs and to feel vulnerable on this trip. With each step you take together, your bond gets stronger and more connected. You can look forward to brighter days and enjoy the journey itself by concentrating on love, empathy, and hope.

Chapter 6

Restoring Intimacy and Romance

It takes both emotional and physical intimacy to rekindle passion and intimacy in a relationship. Building a relationship based on trust, enjoyment, and understanding is what true intimacy is all about, not just physical contact. This chapter will discuss how to re-establish and strengthen intimacy through modest gestures of affection, emotional attachment, and patience as you get to know one another better.

Developing Emotional Closeness
Beyond Physical Intimacy There are other ways to feel connected to one another outside physical closeness, which is a unique aspect of any love relationship. Emotional intimacy is frequently the cornerstone of a solid and fulfilling relationship and can be equally potent. Being able to express ideas, emotions, and dreams without worrying about criticism is a sign of emotional

intimacy. It all comes down to your partner making you feel important, connected, and supported.

1. **Share Your Dreams and Goals with your Partner**

Both partners can feel more connected in each other's lives when they discuss their aspirations, ambitions, and hopes. By expressing these individual goals, you create a strong emotional bond and demonstrate that you are a group with common goals for the future. Schedule time for both solo and couple conversations about your goals and what brings you joy. It might take place over a laid-back evening or over a peaceful meal. This honesty strengthens your emotional connection.

2. **Engage In activities that Make you Happy**:

Engaging in enjoyable activities can foster a playful bond, deepening emotional intimacy. Shared activities, like taking a stroll, watching a movie, or exploring a new hobby, let both spouses unwind while spending time together. Pick something you both like to do or try something new together.
The intention is to foster happy, humorous, and companionable moments to strengthen your bond.

3. **Together, We Are Vulnerable:**

Sharing your pleasures, worries, and concerns is a sign of vulnerability. Vulnerability is a potent technique to increase emotional connection, even though it could initially feel frightening. By being transparent, you demonstrate your mutual trust, which can foster a secure and encouraging environment in your partnership. Encourage your companion to share tiny, intimate thoughts or feelings first. When vulnerable, you feel closer and more connected because it promotes empathy and understanding. A solid basis for intimacy is created by emotional closeness, which gives both partners a sense of security, support, and worth in the partnership.

4. **Embrace Affection**

The tiniest gestures of affection can occasionally have the greatest effects. These small actions let your spouse know that you value them, that you're thinking about them, and that you care. It's typically the little things that provide the most warmth and happiness to a relationship; small acts of love don't need big planning or extravagant displays.

5. **Words of Confirmation:**

It takes a lot of kind words to make someone feel loved. A simple "I love you" or words of gratitude can make your partner's day and deepen your relationship. Your relationship can feel warm and happy if you openly express your affection for your partner, acknowledge their strengths, or thank them for their support. Make an effort to mention one nice thing to your significant other every day. It could be a straightforward way to show your gratitude, something they accomplished, or a trait you find admirable.

6. **Contemplative Surprises**:
Surprises don't have to be costly to have a significant effect. You can tell them you're thinking of them with tiny actions like making their favorite snack, sending a sweet note, or offering a modest sign of affection. Your lover will feel loved and appreciated if you give them thoughtful surprises. Put a small note in your partner's luggage, the bathroom mirror, or somewhere else they'll find it. It's a straightforward approach to make them smile and improve their day.

7. **Acts of Generosity**:
Assisting one another with minor chores demonstrates your concern and wants to lighten your day. Small gestures of kindness, such as helping out around the

house, making breakfast, or offering assistance when they're busy, can foster a caring and supportive environment. Offer to assist with a task they often complete, such as cooking or cleaning. Your companion may feel supported and cared for by this simple gesture of affection.

8. **Physical Love:**

Holding hands, embracing, or gently touching someone are examples of non-sexual physical affection that can foster a feeling of comfort and intimacy. Physical contact is a potent means of expressing love and support without using words. While watching a show, try holding hands or giving each other a few more prolonged hugs. These small gestures demonstrate love and deepen the emotional connection. Every day may be made happier and more connected with small gestures of affection. These actions foster a loving and supportive connection by letting your partner know they are appreciated and adored.

How to Develop Comfort and Trust:

It takes time to rekindle closeness and romance. It takes time, understanding, and a dedication to mutual growth to establish trust and create a welcoming environment.

Knowing that you are both prepared to make an effort to help, listen, and stick by each other's sides fosters comfort and trust.

1. **Having patience with one another**: It's normal to desire answers to problems as soon as possible, yet hurrying can occasionally lead to needless tension. Restoring intimacy and trust requires patience. Recognize that rekindling romance is a process that cannot be rushed, and give each other time to mature and adapt. Let each other know that it's acceptable to take your time. Patience fosters a safe environment where both partners feel at ease by respecting one another's sentiments.

2. **Promoting Open Communication:** Openness and honesty are the foundations of trust. Encourage one another to express their ideas, emotions, and worries without worrying about being judged. Communicating openly demonstrates your mutual respect for one another's viewpoints and readiness to listen. Develop the practice of regularly checking in with one another. "How are you feeling?" ask, or "Are you thinking about anything?" These brief enquiries demonstrate your concern and desire to comprehend one another.

3. **Establishing a Feeling of Safety**:

In any relationship, both partners must feel safe and comfortable. Creating a supportive environment entails supporting one another through happy and difficult times. Knowing that your partner will always be there for you can be consoling, and it might deepen your emotional connection.

Assure one another that you are dedicated to resolving the issue together. Simple phrases like "We'll get through this together" or "I'm here for you" can reassure and reassure.

4. **Taking Advantage of Silent:**

Times Together It's not necessary to be active or talkative all the time. Sometimes, a profound sense of comfort can be created by enjoying each other's company in peaceful moments. These quiet times can promote a sense of connection and tranquility, whether spent sipping tea together, lounging on the couch, or taking in a sunset.

Schedule unscheduled time to spend together. Let's just enjoy one other's company, be together, and feel the warmth of companionship throughout these moments. A solid basis for reigniting romance is established by comfort, patience, and trust. It's simpler to increase closeness and relish the process of getting closer when both parties feel protected, appreciated, and secure.

Accepting a New Phase of Personal Relationships

A continuous process that incorporates both emotional and physical connection is rekindling romance and intimacy. You can establish a relationship based on love, respect, and understanding by developing emotional intimacy, engaging in tiny acts of kindness, and encouraging patience and trust. Keep in mind that intimacy is more than simply a physical relationship; it's also about being there for one another, enjoying each other's company, and developing a safe and encouraging relationship. Every action you perform together contributes to creating a warm, cozy, and profoundly connected relationship.

Let every day be a time to strengthen your bond, encourage one another, and relish the process of reigniting your romance as you welcome this new chapter in your relationship. You're building a love that endures no matter what obstacles you face, whether by kindness, laughing, or peaceful companionship.

Chapter 7

When to Seek Professional Assistance

Sometimes, a little more help is needed to overcome obstacles in relationships or health. Although getting professional assistance can be frightening, doing so is a vital first step towards a more solid and healthy partnership. Seeking help for emotional or interpersonal difficulties can offer relief, direction, and hope, much as when you go to the doctor for a physical injury. In this chapter, we'll discuss why asking for help is OK, how to do it, and how to collaborate as a team throughout the process. Recall that asking for assistance is normal and that working together to take this step can be a constructive way to proceed. Everyone experiences hardships, and although self-help methods are helpful, there are instances in which expert advice might be crucial.

Consulting a therapist, counsellor, or other mental health professional can offer new skills, new insights, and a secure environment for overcoming obstacles.

1. **Eliminating Stigma**:

Many people believe they should be able to manage everything independently and are ashamed or reluctant to ask for assistance. However, in practice, relationship and mental health issues are equally as significant as physical ones, and seeking help is never a sign of weakness. Asking for assistance demonstrates your strength and dedication to enhancing your relationship and general well-being. Remember that asking for assistance is expected, and many people rely on experts to help them through challenging times. Asking for help is not a sign of weakness; on the contrary, it is a step towards recovery and development.

2. **Understanding When Assistance Is Needed**

Determining when professional assistance is necessary might be challenging, particularly if you're accustomed to handling problems alone. If you're dealing with persistent stress, trouble communicating, or severe emotional difficulties, it might be time to consider getting in touch.

Among the indicators that could be helpful are Persistent or intense depressive, anxious, or frustrated feelings and the Inability to adequately communicate with one another. Unresolved problems or ongoing conflict in the relationship – Handling Physical signs of stress, such as headaches or exhaustion: Pay attention to how you feel. If, despite your best efforts, nothing seems to be getting better, it can indicate that you need expert treatment.

3. **Support Types Offered**:
Professionals of many kinds can assist with personal and relationship difficulties.

Essential Aspects to consider when seeking Assistance:

Consult a Counsellor and Therapists:
Counselors are trained to assist with emotional and interpersonal problems. They can provide insightful advice and practical techniques to enhance communication, settle disputes, and control stress.

Consult Health experts:

Physicians or experts can offer diagnoses, treatments, and individualized guidance for physical health issues that impact intimacy.

Join Support groups:
Connecting with people going through similar things can occasionally be beneficial. Support groups offer a secure environment for learning, sharing, and finding solace in knowing you're not alone. Spend some time learning about the kind of help that suits you best. Finding the right counselor or therapist is crucial, but many begin with one focusing on relationships.

Locating the Right Therapist and Consultant

Selecting the appropriate expert might make all the difference once you're ready to ask for assistance. Here's how to get your search started and feel secure about your decision:

1. **Request Suggestions**

Ask people you know who have had good experiences with counseling or therapy for recommendations. You can also locate reliable experts through friends, relatives, or even internet evaluations.

Additionally, your primary care physician might be able to refer mental health providers or other resources. Advice: Never be afraid to ask for help from the people you can trust in your life. Numerous people can offer insightful advice on locating a suitable counselor or support group because they have experienced similar circumstances.

2. **Seek out Experience in Your Field:** Relationship problems or specific health difficulties are the areas of expertise for some therapists and counselors. When looking into your choices, try to find someone who has dealt with the problems you are encountering before. More pertinent resources and insights from a therapist specializing in relationship counseling or health-related issues are frequently available. You may quickly identify the topics each therapist focuses on by looking at the specializations listed on many professional websites. Seek experts who address relationship health, stress reduction, or other issues pertinent to your needs.

3. **Make sure you're at ease:** Since trust is a crucial component of effective counseling, it is imperative that you feel at ease with the professional you select. Many therapists provide a free initial visit to give you a sense of their approach and style. Select someone who gives you a

sense of support, respect, and being heard. Advice: Until you locate the proper specialist, don't be scared to try a few different ones. Establishing a good and trustworthy relationship with your counselor is worth the extra work.

Although asking for assistance can seem significant, getting the correct support can lead to short-term respite and long-term development.

When both parties are on the same page, seeking assistance becomes a collaborative experience that improves the relationship. Working as a team entails being there for one another, listening honestly, and encouraging one another at every stage.

How to Go About Seeking Professional Assistance:

1. **Establishing Common Objectives:** Talking about what you both expect to achieve from counseling or assistance facilitates aligning your attention. Do you both want deeper understanding, better communication, or detailed guidance on how to deal with stress?

Establishing common objectives gives the process focus and a sense of purpose. It's a good idea to spend a few minutes discussing your expectations. Working together to understand one another's aspirations can foster a strong sense of teamwork, even if your aims are slightly different.

2. **Supporting One Another's Emotions:** Counselling can trigger feelings or perhaps reveal problems you may not have been aware were bothering you. We must stand by one another at difficult times. Encourage transparency, listen to one another's emotions, and provide comfort. Understanding and acknowledging one another's experiences facilitates building comfort and trust.

Tip: After every session, check in with one another. "How are you feeling?" or "Is there anything you want to discuss? These little actions demonstrate support and give each partner a sense of being heard and understood.

2. **Honouring Advancements**
No Matter How Minor, Not all growth occurs rapidly. Even if some changes will be gradual, any little advancement is cause for celebration. You can maintain your

motivation and optimism about the journey by noticing minor gains, such as feeling more at ease or speaking more freely.

Tip: Take the time to acknowledge one another's advancements. Any progress, no matter how small, should be accepted. When using positive reinforcement, the procedure can seem pleasant and promote further development.

Maintaining Patience as a Top Concern

Resolving issues and strengthening your bond takes time. Patience is crucial when navigating both the good and the bad days. By showing each other patience, you reaffirm that you are in this together and are prepared to give each other the space and time they require to recover and develop.

Tip: Let each other know that it's acceptable to proceed cautiously. Even when things seem moving slowly, patience makes you feel valued and supported.

Seeking professional treatment indicates that you care enough to invest in the health of your relationship, not that there is something "wrong" with you or it. Professionals provide the direction and assistance required for emotional and relational well-being, much like we see doctors for physical health. Approaching it collectively turns it into a team endeavor to develop a deeper understanding of one another and create a solid, enduring bond. Keep in mind that every step forward is an indication of strength rather than weakness. It shows your commitment and love when you ask for help together. You're taking a significant step towards a more contented and connected relationship by cooperating, listening to one another, and acknowledging your accomplishments.

Conclusion

Advancing Together

As this voyage comes to a close, remember that each step you've taken has led to a closer, more solid partnership. Rekindling intimacy, healing, and growth are gradual processes interspersed with moments of love, patience, and understanding. In the same way, you have overcome obstacles together, you may keep constructing a future based on grit, optimism, and intimacy.

Recognize Little Achievements:
Every little victory counts in life, and they should all be celebrated. A meaningful talk, a vulnerable moment, or a constructive shift in how you support one another are all indications of growth. When thinking about the big picture, it's simple to miss these little victories, but acknowledging them can make your journey happier and more motivating. Little victories serve as a reminder that even the most minor progress matters. They build

up to a more satisfying, affectionate connection over time. Thus, remember to stop, acknowledge, and appreciate every small step forward. Let these moments serve as a source of pride and inspiration to keep going, whether it's a thoughtful act, a novel approach to managing stress, or just a sense of closeness. Develop the practice of sharing in minor triumphs. It might be as easy as spending a peaceful evening together or expressing gratitude. You will feel more motivated to continue developing as a team the more you celebrate these occasions.

A Stronger and Closer Future:
You've learned from this voyage that obstacles are only chances for personal development. You've made significant progress towards a resilient and connected relationship by emphasizing a comprehensive approach that nurtures physical and emotional well-being. As you move forward, remember that every experience—no matter how positive or challenging—brings you closer and fortifies your relationship. Continue to foster open communication, show patience to one another, and take delight in the small things in life.

Although there will always be ups and downs, you have established a foundation to withstand those times together. Embrace the future with optimism and hope, knowing you both have what it takes to create a successful partnership. A lovely, continuous trip is just getting started. Every day is an opportunity to deepen your relationship, encourage one another, and spend time together. Remain optimistic, continue to develop as a team, and never forget that the best is still to come and that you are more potent when you are unified. I appreciate you traveling this path with me.

Cheers to a future full of love, strength, and the delight of genuine connection…

9 7 9 8 3 0 2 0 5 4 4 6 3